HEART-HEALTHY COOKBOOK FOR BEGINNERS

"Transform Your Heart Health With 2000+ Days of Delicious Recipes to Low-Fat, Blood Pressure and Cholesterol Level. Include a 60-Day Meal Plan and Professional Advice for Optimal Health"

VICTOR WREN

COPYRIGHT © 2024 BY VICTOR WREN

ABSTRACT

The **"Heart Healthy Cookbook for Beginners"** provides an essential culinary guide perfectly tailored for those dedicated to nurturing a heart-friendly lifestyle. Bursting with an array of diverse and delicious recipes, this extensive manual covers a wide spectrum of culinary traditions and dietary preferences.

It explores core cooking methods, emphasizing wholesome and well-rounded meals while considering various dietary limitations. Promoting mindful consumption, it encourages savoring every morsel.

This guide is a repository of practical guidance, empowering both newcomers and seasoned chefs with flexible recipes, enriching their understanding of heart-conscious eating. Above all, it stands as an invaluable companion, igniting inspiration and guiding individuals on a flavorful and heart-aware culinary voyage.

TABLE OF CONTENTS

-Integrating Heart-Healthy Habits into Hectic Schedules
-Navigating Heart-Conscious Grocery Shopping

Chapter Four:
Special Dietary Adjustments
-Welcoming Dietary Variance
-Elevating Flavor without Sacrifice
-Tips on maintaining taste and flavor while making dietary adjustments

Chapter Five:
Creating Your Essential Heart-Healthy Pantry
-Comprehensive list of staple ingredients for a heart-healthy kitchen
-Organizational tips for keeping the pantry well-stocked and efficient

Chapter Six:
60-Day Meal Plan
-60-Day meal plan with diverse, flavorful, and easy-to-follow recipes
-Balanced Breakfast Ideas
-Nutrient-Packed Lunches
-Wholesome Dinner Delights
-Smart and Healthy Snack Choices
-Daily Guidance and Timely Schedules

-Detailed daily schedules to guide beginners through the meal plan

Chapter Seven: FAQ Highlights
-Addressing common questions about heart-healthy cooking
-Troubleshooting guide for beginner cooks facing challenges in the kitchen

Chapter Eight:
2000+ Days of Diverse Recipes
-A vast selection of over 2000 recipes spanning various cuisines and flavors
-Categorization based on meal types, ingredients, and cooking difficulty levels
-Emphasis on variety to keep meals exciting and enjoyable

Chapter Nine: Conclusion
-Summarizing the key takeaways from the cookbook
-Encouragement and motivation for readers to continue their journey toward heart-healthy cooking
-Closing remarks and best wishes for a healthier lifestyle

Appendix

INTRODUCTION

The **Heart Healthy Cookbook for Beginners** isn't just a recipe collection; it's an invitation to embrace heart-conscious eating as a fundamental aspect of overall wellness.

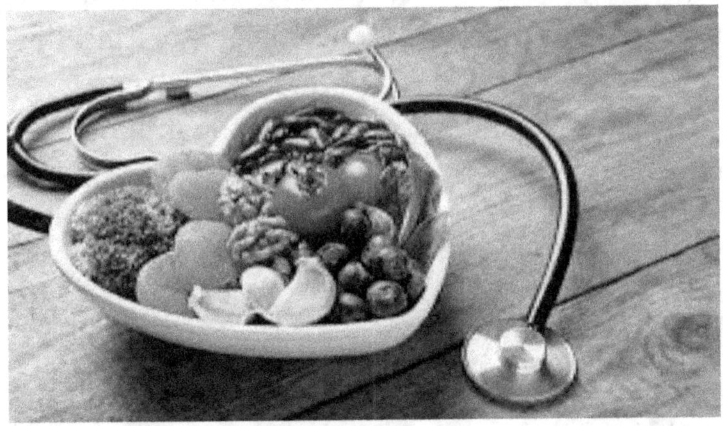

Tailored for beginners, this guide promises an accessible and enjoyable journey into heart-healthy cooking, regardless of kitchen expertise.

Beyond recipes, it fosters a connection between nourishment, heart health, and shared experiences. Offering simple culinary practices, insights on heart health, and practical tips, it aims to create a meaningful relationship with well-being through food. It encourages readers to immerse themselves in kitchen adventures, connecting with a community on a similar path toward a healthier, more fulfilling life.

Cheers to vibrant health and delightful culinary discoveries!

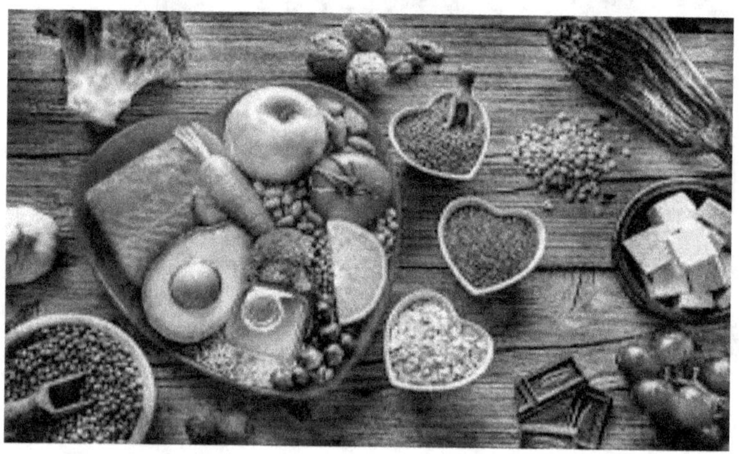

CHAPTER ONE
COOKING MADE SIMPLE

Welcome to the doorway of culinary expertise! In this chapter, we embark on a voyage that simplifies the craft of cooking, making it accessible and enjoyable for all newcomers venturing into the realm of heart-healthy cuisine.

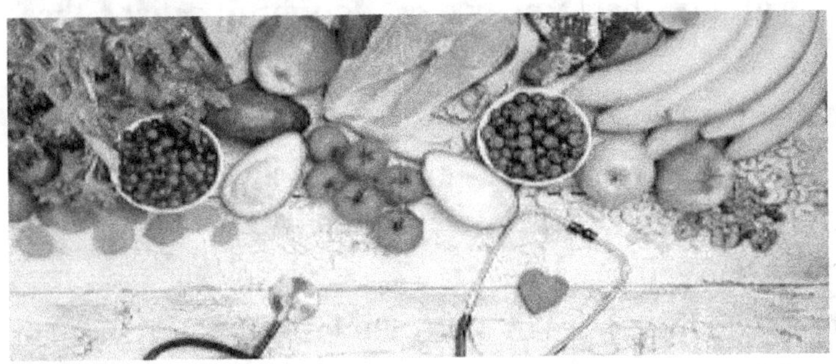

1:1. MASTERING ESSENTIAL COOKING TECHNIQUES

1. Mastering Key Culinary Methods:

The cultivation of culinary skill relies on the mastery of fundamental techniques that lay the groundwork for creating extraordinary dishes. Within this section, we embark on an illuminating exploration into the core culinary methodologies crucial for fashioning delectable and heart-healthy meals.

2. Understanding the Basics: Culinary Approaches

Cooking methods serve as the artisan's brushstrokes on the canvas of gastronomy. Each approach triggers a distinctive metamorphosis in ingredients, unlocking a symphony of flavors, textures, and fragrances. From the delicate finesse of poaching, which retains tenderness, to the scorching intensity of grilling that imparts a delightful char, these methods define the essence of culinary craftsmanship.

3. Delving into Intricacies: Techniques Unveiled

Delve deeper into the intricacies inherent in each technique. Unearth the artistry of sautéing, where ingredients pirouette in the pan, acquiring a golden hue and delicate essence. Uncover the alchemical process of braising, where slow cooking in liquid tenderizes tough portions, yielding succulent, mouthwatering sensations.

4. **Achieving Equilibrium: Balancing Flavors and Textures**

Mastering these techniques transcends mere adherence to instructions; it involves orchestrating a harmonious interplay of tastes and sensations. Explore how roasting amplifies flavors, caramelizing natural sugars to craft a richness that captivates the palate. Dive into the nuances of steaming, which conserves nutrients and generates dishes bursting with vibrant freshness.

5. **Going Beyond Recipes: Fostering Culinary Ingenuity**

Comprehending these foundational methods bestows upon you the liberty to innovate. Armed with this knowledge, you're liberated from the confines of recipes, guided instead by an awareness of how heat, time, and technique mold the outcome of your culinary endeavors.

6. Confidence in the Kitchen: Honing Techniques

Embrace practice as your ally. Experiment, adapt, and refine these techniques until they become an innate skill. Through hands-on experience, you'll amass the confidence to wield these culinary tools effortlessly, transforming raw ingredients into masterpieces that not only tantalize taste buds but also nurture the soul.

By mastering these pivotal culinary techniques, you embark on a journey transcending recipes, assuming the role of the architect of your culinary journey. Through comprehension, practice, and innovation, you unlock the gateway to a realm where every dish serves as a canvas for your culinary expression.

1:2. KNIFE SKILLS WITH PRECISION

1. Perfecting Knife Craft: Mastery in Blade Handling

Mastery in culinary expertise necessitates a thorough exploration into the finesse of maneuvering a blade. This section delves into the art of refining knife skills, elevating them beyond mere chopping to embody precision and absolute control within the culinary domain.

2. Grasping the Craft: Proficiency in Knife Handling

Efficient knife handling surpasses basic cutting; it embodies a fusion of precision and authority. This exploration delves deep into the anatomy of the blade, unraveling its complexities and acknowledging its pivotal role in mastering culinary finesse.

3. Journey into Cutting Techniques: An Odyssey through Precision

Embark on a voyage to master an array of cutting methods, uncovering the artistry within each technique. From the graceful slice to the meticulous julienne, each movement is meticulously crafted to metamorphose ingredients into culinary wonders. This immersion fosters a comprehensive understanding of how varied cuts enrich both the aesthetics and flavors of your culinary creations.

4. Enhancing Culinary Expertise: Streamlined Efficiency and Safety

Enhancing blade finesse not only expedites meal preparation but also guarantees safety and heightens the visual allure of your culinary palette. Embrace techniques that not only streamline your cooking process but also elevate the overall artistic presentation of heart-healthy ingredients.

5. Precision as Culinary Expression: Visual Elegance

Precision in knife skills serves as a distinct dialect within the culinary lexicon. Every incision, slice, or chop is a statement, crafting not just food but an artistic display that entices the eyes before tantalizing the taste buds.

6. Embracing Proficiency through Repeated Practice: The Road to Mastery

Welcome practice as your companion on the quest to master knife skills. Engage in consistent practice, allowing these skills to evolve from conscious actions to intuitive maneuvers. Through dedicated repetition and refinement, transform blade handling into an innate and seamless facet of your culinary repertoire.

Hone your knife skills with precision, unlocking a realm where blade mastery transcends mere culinary technique, evolving into a form of culinary finesse that infuses sophistication, safety, and efficacy into your culinary masterpieces.

1:3. EFFICIENT TIME MANAGEMENT AND CULINARY TIPS

1. Optimizing Time and Culinary Insights

In the culinary arena, harnessing time efficiently stands as vital as mastering flavors. This section plunges into the domain of effective time utilization and culinary sagacity, furnishing you with invaluable methodologies to maximize your kitchen hours while augmenting the excellence and relish of your heart-healthy culinary masterpieces.

2. Strategic Time Management: Crafting Kitchen Efficiency

Efficiency within the kitchen orchestrates a nuanced harmony between groundwork and execution. Unearth methodologies to arrange and streamline your cooking trajectory, ensuring every moment spent resonates with purpose and productivity. From prepping ingredients beforehand to orchestrating multifaceted culinary maneuvers, discover techniques that capitalize on your precious kitchen moments without compromising taste or nutritional value.

3. Time-Economizing Culinary Strategies: Clever Expedients

Embark on a trove of resourceful tips and crafty shortcuts aimed at saving time without compromising on culinary quality. From astute shortcuts for precision chopping and slicing to maximizing the efficacy of kitchen tools, these tricks pledge to revolutionize your culinary journey. Unveil methodologies that expedite meal preparation while preserving the essence of heart-healthy ingredients, enabling the creation of savory dishes with efficiency.

4. Strategic Meal Planning: Beyond Batch Cooking

Immerse yourself in the art of strategic meal planning and the realm of batch cooking, indispensable tools in the repertoire of an efficient chef. Discover how deliberate planning and preparation can yield multiple meals from a single cooking session. Reveal the advantages of batch cooking, allowing you to stock your freezer with nourishing, ready-to-indulge meals, curtailing cooking time on bustling days while relishing in wholesome homemade dishes.

5. Efficiency in Tidiness: Organizational Tips

Efficiency transcends the culinary sphere—it encompasses orderliness and structure. Explore methodologies to sustain an organized kitchen, facilitating smoother cooking experiences. Unearth insights for decluttering, optimizing storage, and preserving a pristine workspace, ensuring each culinary endeavor commences and culminates with efficiency and convenience.

6. Harmonizing Speed with Quality: The Culinary Equilibrium

Efficient time management need not compromise the quality or relish of your culinary creations. Strike a harmonious equilibrium between promptness and culinary brilliance. Reveal techniques ensuring that, even amidst time constraints, your heart-healthy creations endure as flavorful, nourishing, and visually captivating.

7. Savoring the Fruits: Efficiency and Epicurean Contentment

Effective time management within the kitchen becomes a gateway to culinary contentment. By mastering these time-saving methodologies and culinary ingenuity, you not only optimize your cooking hours but also elevate your culinary finesse, permitting you to revel in the outcomes of efficient, delectable, and heart-healthy homemade meals.

1:4. INTRODUCTION TO ESSENTIAL KITCHEN TOOLS AND THEIR USES

Efficiently navigating the culinary realm requires a comprehensive grasp of and proficiency in wielding foundational kitchen implements. This section acts as your portal into the realm of vital kitchen apparatus, unraveling their significance and the wide-ranging applications they possess in curating appetizing, heart-healthy meals.

1. Understanding the Kitchen Arsenal: Instruments and Their Functions

The operational efficiency of a kitchen is intricately linked to the array of tools it houses. Dive into the spectrum of utensils, devices, and machinery that constitute the backbone of culinary pursuits. From the unassuming wooden spatula to the versatile chef's knife, each implement serves a distinct role, contributing indispensably to a seamless cooking narrative.

2. In-depth Analysis of Essential Tools: Disclosing Utility

Explore the detailed structure and utility of essential kitchen implements. Uncover the intricacies of their design, ergonomic attributes, and distinctive functionalities that render each tool indispensable. Gain a profound understanding of how these implements facilitate tasks such as mincing, stirring, emulsifying, gauging, and cooking, empowering you to wield them with exactitude and efficacy.

3. Versatile Adaptability: Tools Tailored for Varied Functions

Witness firsthand the versatility inherent in kitchen implements, surpassing singular purposes to cater to a myriad of culinary requirements. Examine how a simple spatula transcends flipping to stirring and scraping, or how a mixing bowl metamorphoses from a vessel for amalgamating ingredients into a platform for kneading dough or marinating meats.

4. Instruments for Precision and Expertise: Elevation of Culinary Mastery

Recognize how the apt choice of tools augments culinary finesse and exactness. Observe how a finely honed paring knife facilitates intricate slicing, while a robust whisk metamorphoses ingredients into aeration excellence. Each implement, when adeptly wielded, evolves into an extension of culinary expertise, heightening both the efficiency and artistry of the culinary endeavor.

5. Foundational Kitchen Elements: Cornerstones of Culinary Ingenuity

Appreciate these kitchen implements not just as tools but as catalysts for culinary ingenuity. They lay the groundwork for experimentation and innovation, providing budding chefs with the canvas to experiment, adapt, and compose an assortment of enticing dishes.

6. Proficiency through Familiarity: Embracing Mastery of Implements

Embrace familiarity with these implements as the bedrock of culinary adeptness. Through practice, comprehension, and familiarity, transform the handling of these tools from mechanical maneuvers into intuitive actions, amplifying your culinary repertoire and fostering a profounder connection between your culinary vision and the implements at your disposal.

Embark on an exploration through the pivotal implements of the kitchen, where each tool becomes a catalyst for culinary creativity, transforming raw constituents into tantalizing dishes that not only gratify the palate but also mirror the finesse and craftsmanship of the chef.

Equip yourself through this chapter with the foundational knowledge essential to commence a culinary journey marked by ease, efficacy, and newfound confidence in your culinary skills. As we unravel the intricacies of techniques, tools, and time-saving methods, prepare to metamorphose your kitchen into a space where heart-healthy creations flourish effortlessly, one delectable dish at a time.

CHAPTER TWO

FOCUSED GUIDANCE FOR HEART HEALTH

Delving into the realm of heart vitality necessitates a holistic grasp of core aspects, deliberate decision-making, and the cultivation of mindful lifestyle habits. This segment stands as your guiding beacon, escorting you through the intricate dimensions of fostering a heart-healthy existence.

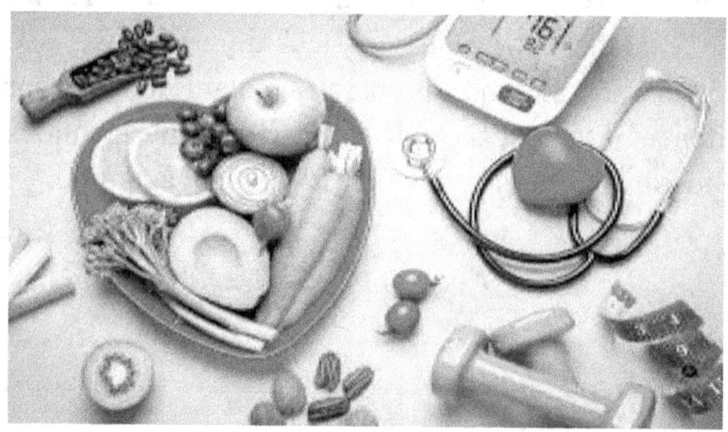

2:1. EXPLORATION OF HEART-HEALTHY INGREDIENTS:
UNVEILING BENEFITS

1. Journeying Through Heart-Enhancing Ingredients: Unveiling Their Merits

Embarking on an immersive quest into heart-friendly ingredients unveils a trove of nutritional advantages and health benefits. This expedition brings to light the distinctive attributes of specific elements that profoundly contribute to fortifying and nurturing cardiovascular well-being.

2. Revealing the Nutritional Abundance: Grasping Their Vital Importance

This exploration reveals the inherent richness of nutrients present in heart-healthy ingredients, highlighting their essential functions in bolstering heart health. Unveil the abundance of vitamins, minerals, and antioxidants housed within these elements, illustrating their ability to strengthen and protect the heart from potential illnesses and threats.

3. Empowering Heart Health: Leveraging Their Therapeutic Qualities

Beyond their nutritional essence, these heart-empowering ingredients boast therapeutic potentials. Delve deeper into their medicinal virtues, witnessing their active contribution to maintaining optimal blood pressure, cholesterol equilibrium, and overall cardiac functionality. From their anti-inflammatory attributes to their role in augmenting blood vessel resilience, these constituents emerge as holistic guardians of heart wellness.

4. Foundational Elements for Heart Resilience: Vital Ingredients for Well-being

Comprehend the pivotal role these ingredients play as the bedrock of heart robustness. They serve as the keystones for crafting a heart-conscious dietary framework, their multifaceted advantages nurturing a durable cardiovascular system. Ranging from the omega-3 fatty acids prevalent in fish to the phytonutrients abundant in vibrant fruits and vegetables, these constituents fortify the heart against potential health hazards.

5. Achieving Holistic Wellness: Harmonizing Health through Ingredients

This expedition not only reveals their individual merits but also unveils the synergy these ingredients bring to a holistic dietary approach. Acknowledge their capacity to elevate overall well-being while particularly targeting heart health. Observe how integrating them into daily meals fosters a comprehensive nourishment strategy, culminating in a vigorous and flourishing cardiovascular system.

Peeling back the layers of heart-boosting ingredients through this expansive journey unveils their diverse benefits and pivotal role in fortifying heart wellness. Embrace this knowledge as a cornerstone for sculpting a nourishing and heart-conscious dietary lifestyle.

2:2. UNDERSTANDING FOOD IMPACT ON HEART HEALTH:

THE CULINARY INFLUENCE

Delving into the correlation between our food intake and heart well-being reveals the substantial influence our dietary selections wield. This comprehensive investigation navigates the complex interactions within our diets and cardiovascular vitality.

Explore the intricate impacts of diverse nutrients, fats, sugars, and dietary constituents, unraveling their significant ramifications on heart health.

Enjoy uncovering the ways certain foods impact cholesterol levels, regulate blood pressure, and contribute to overall heart functionality, fostering a profound comprehension that facilitates proactive choices in formulating a heart-supportive dietary regimen.

2:3. SIGNIFICANCE OF PORTION CONTROL AND MINDFUL EATING HABITS : BALANCING WELLNESS

Appreciating the importance of managing portion sizes and integrating mindfulness into eating habits plays a fundamental role in nurturing a well-rounded and healthy way of life.

Embrace the essence of controlling portion sizes and incorporating mindfulness into meal consumption, cultivating a sense of equilibrium and wellness within your dietary routine.

These methodologies not only assist in weight management but also foster a more profound relationship with the food you consume, resulting in a more fulfilling and health-oriented eating journey.

This targeted counsel intertwines the exploration of heart-enriching elements, the comprehension of food's influence on heart health, and the cultivation of mindful eating practices. It stands as a guiding force on your path toward a heart-aware lifestyle, empowering you to make judicious dietary decisions and foster practices that fortify a resilient and vibrant heart.

CHAPTER THREE

PRACTICAL INSIGHTS FOR DAILY HEART-HEALTHY COOKING

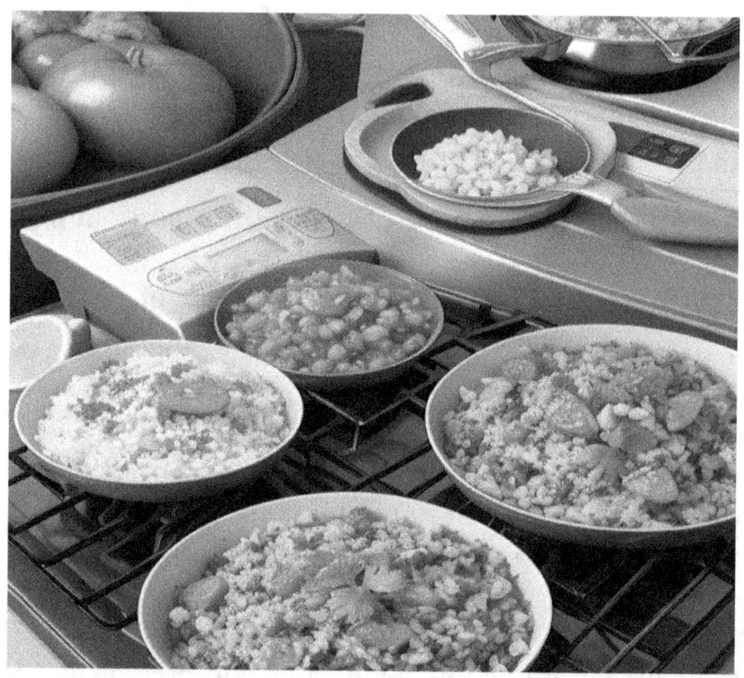

3:1. MASTERING MEAL PREPARATION AND PLANNING STRATEGIES

Unearth effective methodologies for meal prepping and planning, fundamental pillars in effortlessly integrating heart-healthy meals into your routine.

Discover the artistry of preparing meals ahead, streamlining your time management, and establishing a range of nutritious choices easily accessible throughout your week.

Acquire the skill to design adaptable meal plans, empowering you to navigate hectic schedules while steadfastly pursuing your heart-conscious dietary aspirations.

1. Development of a Meal Preparation Framework

Embark on the journey of crafting an efficient meal preparation framework tailored to your dietary inclinations and daily agenda. Acquire the knack for identifying recipes that adhere to heart-healthy guidelines while satisfying your palate. Cultivate a methodical approach to meal planning, emphasizing nutritional equilibrium, diversity, and simplicity in meal assembly.

2. Techniques for Optimizing Time

Unearth strategies to streamline meal preparation without compromising quality or flavor. Explore methodologies to enhance efficiency, including batch cooking, leveraging kitchen appliances ingeniously, and orchestrating simultaneous tasks during culinary preparation. These approaches transform meal preparation into a manageable and time-efficient endeavor.

3. Adaptable Meal Plans for Dynamic Lifestyles

Curate flexible meal plans adaptable to the ever-changing rhythm of everyday life. Recognize the significance of adaptability in meal planning, enabling alterations while upholding heart-healthy principles. Embrace versatility in meal selections, ensuring seamless integration into diverse schedules and routines.

4. Organizational Tactics for Meal Excellence

Acquire insights into organizational strategies fostering success in meal preparation. Uncover tips for expedient grocery shopping, savvy ingredient storage, and pragmatic kitchen arrangement. A well-organized culinary environment streamlines meal preparation, fostering a consistent routine in crafting heart-healthy dishes.

5. Long-term Sustainability in Meal Design

Explore sustainable practices in meal planning, emphasizing the creation of a durable and viable approach. Strike a harmonious balance between variety, ease of execution, and nutritional value, ensuring the long-term sustenance of heart-conscious dietary habits.

Mastery of meal preparation and planning strategies empowers the seamless infusion of heart-healthy culinary creations into your daily regimen. A meticulously devised meal preparation framework, time-saving methodologies, adaptability, organizational finesse, and a focus on sustainability form the bedrock for a journey toward a nourishing and heart-conscious lifestyle.

3:2.   INTEGRATING   HEART-HEALTHY HABITS INTO HECTIC SCHEDULES

Explore pragmatic methods to infuse heart-healthy habits into demanding schedules. Navigate the complexities of a bustling lifestyle by embracing simple yet impactful practices that prioritize heart well-being. Investigate time-efficient cooking techniques and judicious selections that synchronize seamlessly with your timetable, ensuring that nourishing meals seamlessly integrate into your daily routine.

1. Streamlined Heart-Healthy Decisions

Navigate the intricacies of hectic schedules by simplifying heart-healthy choices. Explore straightforward yet impactful practices that resonate with your fast-paced lifestyle. Embrace slight adjustments in dietary choices or exercise routines tailored to your timetable, fostering heart wellness in manageable and attainable ways.

2. Efficient Cooking Methods for Time Optimization

Explore time-saving culinary techniques that complement a packed schedule without compromising on health. Discover quick and nutritious recipes, shortcuts for meal preparation, or effective cooking methods that seamlessly fit into busy days. These methods ensure access to wholesome meals even during the most hectic moments.

3. Infusing Daily Life with Movement

Embrace intermittent physical activity throughout the day. Explore strategies to integrate movement into your routine, whether it's taking short walks during breaks, opting for stairs, or incorporating brief home workouts. These simple activities contribute to overall heart health while blending effortlessly with a bustling schedule.

4. Mindful Stress Alleviation

Explore stress-relieving practices seamlessly integrated into your daily regimen. Discover mindfulness exercises, breathing techniques, or moments of relaxation that aid in managing stress amid hectic schedules. Carving out time for mental rejuvenation supports heart health by lessening the impact of stress.

5. Tailored Self-Care Rituals

Craft personalized self-care rituals that seamlessly merge with your daily grind. Embrace activities that rejuvenate both mind and body, whether it's a few minutes of mindfulness, savoring a nutritious snack deliberately, or finding solace in hobbies. These rituals nurture heart health by fostering overall well-being amid a bustling lifestyle.

Integrating heart-healthy practices into packed schedules involves finding simplicity amid the chaos. By simplifying choices, adopting time-efficient cooking methods, infusing movement, managing stress mindfully, and customizing self-care routines, you pave the way for a heart-conscious lifestyle that seamlessly aligns with your busy routine.

3:3. NAVIGATING HEART-CONSCIOUS GROCERY SHOPPING

Attain guidance on navigating grocery shopping effortlessly to make heart-conscious selections. Master the decoding of food labels, discerning heart-healthy ingredients, and selecting nutritious options while maneuvering through the store aisles. Uncover astute shopping tips that empower you to curate a comprehensive and heart-supportive pantry, ensuring each purchase contributes positively to your overall heart health.

1. Unveiling the Secrets of Nutrition Labels

Sharpen your ability to interpret nutrition labels, a critical skill for informed choices. Dive into ingredient lists, portion sizes, and nutrient details. Master the knack for spotting hidden sugars, unhealthy fats, and excessive sodium, instead opting for options packed with fiber, essential vitamins, and vital nutrients crucial for heart health.

2. Embracing the Bounty of Fresh and Wholesome Foods

Elevate your grocery haul with fresh, nutrient-rich foods. Embrace a cornucopia of colorful fruits, verdant leafy greens, lean proteins, and hearty whole grains—staples that form the bedrock of heart-healthy diets. Explore the vast spectrum of flavors and nutrients these foods offer, enriching both palate and well-being.

3. Crafting Strategic Shopping Plans for Heart Health

Engineer a meticulous shopping blueprint tailored to your heart-conscious aspirations. Design a grocery list aligned with well-rounded nutrition, spotlighting essential ingredients while sidestepping processed and high-sugar choices. Cultivate a diversified array of heart-friendly foods to infuse vitality into your meals.

4. Innovative Exploration of Heart-Healthy Substitutes

Embark on a quest for alternatives that harmonize with heart-conscious dining. Trade out unhealthy options for heart-friendly substitutes: opt for whole-grain goodness, leaner meat cuts, and embrace the world of plant-based proteins. Pave the way for imaginative culinary adventures that blend flavor and texture while nurturing your health.

5. Cultivating a Heart-Nurturing Pantry

Curate a pantry fortified with heart-supporting essentials. Stock up on nuts, seeds, olive oil, legumes, and whole grains—the backbone of heart-conscious culinary endeavors. Transform these staples into versatile ingredients that breathe life into nutritious meals, embodying a fusion of taste and well-being.

Efficiently navigating heart-healthy grocery shopping involves discerning choices that fortify a heart-smart lifestyle.

By deciphering labels, embracing freshness, planning strategically, exploring substitutions, and fostering a heart-nurturing pantry, you lay the groundwork for nourishing meals that become the cornerstone of a vibrant heart and overall health.

This chapter serves as your handbook for intertwining heart-healthy routines into your everyday life.

It furnishes you with practical tactics for meal preparation, accommodating bustling schedules, and making informed decisions during grocery shopping, ensuring that your quest for heart-conscious cooking remains both convenient and enduring.

CHAPTER FOUR

TAILORING FOR DIETARY PREFERENCES

Within this segment, we'll delve into adept adjustments to foster heart-healthy cooking, ensuring it harmonizes with diverse dietary choices without compromising on delightful flavors.

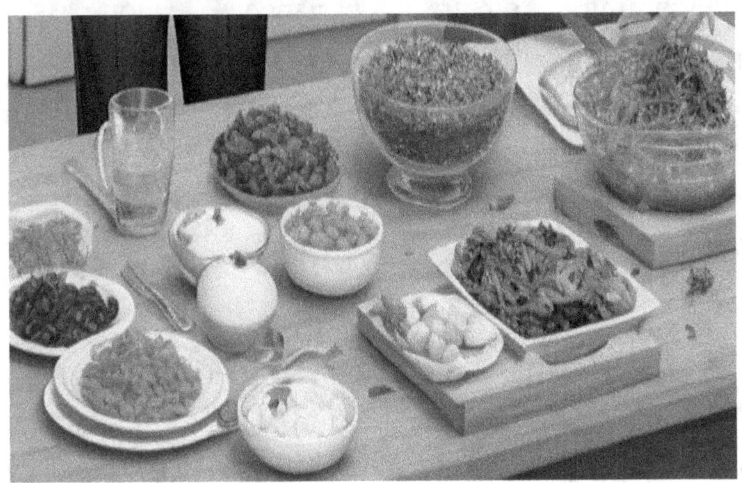

4:1. WELCOMING DIETARY VARIANCE

This chapter offers an exhaustive handbook to embrace an array of dietary preferences. It encompasses guidance for vegan, vegetarian, gluten-free, and other specific dietary needs.

It plunges into the intricacies of modifying recipes, ingredients, and cooking methodologies to align seamlessly with these dietary inclinations. Explore the art of crafting a wide array of heart-healthy dishes tailored to everyone's distinct preferences and nutritional requirements.

1. Grasping Dietary Diversity:

Welcoming dietary variance encompasses understanding the vast range of dietary preferences, encompassing choices such as veganism, vegetarianism, gluten-free diets, and specific allergen considerations. Appreciating the nutritional depth each preference offers involves tailoring meals to suit these varying dietary needs.

2. Adjusting for Unique Requirements:

This exploration delves into the nuances of adapting recipes and meal plans to meet specific dietary needs. It emphasizes the significance of sourcing diverse ingredients, modifying cooking methods, and finding suitable substitutions to craft meals that cater to different dietary choices while upholding their heart-healthy essence.

3. Honoring Culinary Variety:

Embracing dietary variance extends beyond meeting requirements; it involves reveling in the culinary richness each preference brings. This entails exploring novel ingredients, innovative cooking techniques, and a broad spectrum of flavors that complement diverse dietary choices, fostering an inclusive and dynamic culinary journey.

Welcoming dietary variance in heart-healthy cooking fosters an inclusive environment where every dietary preference is acknowledged, understood, and accounted for. It's a testament to recognizing the varied nutritional needs and flavor inclinations of individuals, ensuring that everyone can relish delectable and nutritious meals while supporting heart health.

4:2. ELEVATING FLAVOR WITHOUT SACRIFICE

Preserving taste and flavor while adhering to dietary adjustments is pivotal to an enjoyable dining experience. Uncover methodologies that enhance the flavors of heart-healthy cuisines without infringing upon dietary restrictions. Dive into the world of seasoning amalgamations, culinary techniques, and inventive ingredient pairings that heighten taste profiles and richness, ensuring each dish remains appetizing and captivating.

1. Masterful Seasoning:

The art of crafting delectable heart-healthy meals hinges on mastering seasoning techniques. Dive into the realm of herbs, spices, and unique seasoning blends that infuse depth and richness into dishes. Develop a skill for creatively balancing flavors, creating aromatic profiles that enhance taste without relying on excessive salt or sugar.

2. **Innovative Ingredient Pairings:**
Discover innovative ingredient combinations that elevate taste while respecting various dietary preferences. Experiment with a diverse array of fruits, vegetables, grains, and proteins to concoct enticing flavor unions. Explore how different textures and flavor profiles complement one another, heightening the overall appeal of heart-healthy culinary creations.

3. **Culinary Methods to Amplify Flavor:**
Explore cooking techniques that intensify flavors while maintaining health-conscious standards. Techniques like roasting, grilling, or caramelizing vegetables can heighten their inherent sweetness and robustness. Unveil methods that draw out the natural flavors of ingredients, enhancing the overall taste and appeal of dishes.

Amplifying flavor in heart-healthy cooking involves embracing ingenuity and innovation in the kitchen. By mastering the art of seasoning, experimenting with ingredient pairings, and employing cooking techniques that magnify taste, you'll craft dishes that are not just nutritious but also bursting with an array of delightful flavors.

4:3. TIPS ON MAINTAINING TASTE AND FLAVOR WHILE MAKING DIETARY ADJUSTMENTS

Ensuring that heart-healthy meals remain delicious and fulfilling despite specific dietary needs is crucial. This section presents practical tips and effective strategies to enhance flavors and maintain taste while making necessary dietary adjustments.

1. Embrace the World of Herbs and Spices: Immerse yourself in the vast realm of herbs and spices, elevating your dishes with nuanced depth and intricate flavors. Experiment with a diverse range of seasoning blends, aromatic herbs, and bold spices that elevate taste profiles without resorting to excessive salt, sugar, or unhealthy fats. These elements infuse your meals with a burst of flavor while adhering to various dietary restrictions.

2. Explore the Bounty of Fresh Ingredients:
Dive into a multitude of fresh produce to introduce vibrant and genuine flavors to your cooking. Fruits, vegetables, and herbs not only add taste but also texture and a spectrum of colors to your recipes. Play with a medley of ingredients, incorporating a diverse array of colorful and nutrient-rich components to amplify the sensory experience of your meals.

3. Master the Art of Cooking Techniques:
Discover various cooking methods that intensify flavors while prioritizing health. Techniques such as grilling, roasting, or sautéing bring out the natural essence and textures of ingredients. For instance, roasting vegetables heightens their innate sweetness, while grilling imparts a delightful smokiness, contributing to an elevated culinary journey.

4. Achieve Harmony with Healthy Fats and Acids:

Integrate healthy fats like olive oil, nuts, or avocados to infuse richness and depth into your culinary creations. Similarly, incorporating acidic components like citrus juices, vinegar, or tomatoes lends brightness and a balanced taste profile to your meals, devoid of excessive sodium or processed additives.

5. Embrace Umami's Flavorful Embrace

Incorporate umami-rich elements such as mushrooms, tomatoes, soy sauce, or nutritional yeast to intensify the savory aspects of your recipes. Umami brings a gratifying depth and luxuriousness to dishes, enhancing their flavors and making them more enjoyable, especially in vegetarian or vegan cooking.

By combining a plethora of herbs, fresh produce, diverse cooking methods, healthy fats, acidity, and umami-rich elements, you can enhance and preserve the taste and flavors of heart-healthy meals while seamlessly accommodating various dietary adjustments.

Navigating through unique dietary preferences within the realm of heart-healthy cooking entails an understanding of specific dietary requisites and adapting recipes accordingly.

By presenting an extensive compendium accommodating diverse dietary preferences and providing insights on maintaining taste and flavor during adjustments, this chapter aims to render heart-conscious eating an enjoyable and all-encompassing expedition for all individuals.

CHAPTER FIVE

CREATING YOUR ESSENTIAL HEART-HEALTHY PANTRY

Constructing a heart-conscious kitchen begins with a fully stocked pantry. This section lays out an extensive checklist of crucial elements necessary for crafting nutritious, heart-supporting meals.

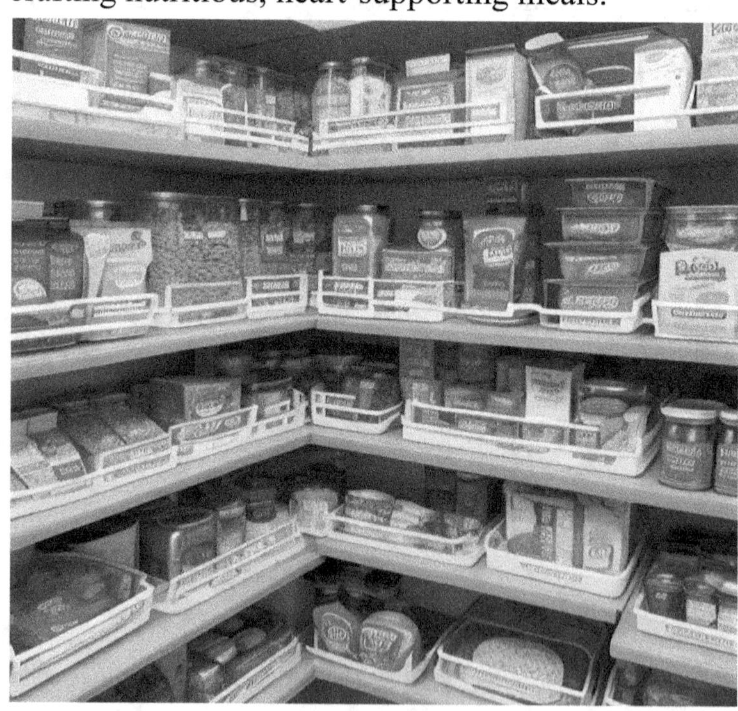

5:1. COMPREHENSIVE LIST OF STAPLE INGREDIENTS FOR A HEART-HEALTHY KITCHEN

1. Whole Grains and Legumes:

> **Quinoa:** Abundant in protein and fiber.
> **Brown Rice:** Nutrient-packed and adaptable.
> **Oats:** Fiber-rich, perfect for breakfast or baking.
> **Lentils:** Protein-rich legumes, ideal for soups and salads.
> **Beans**: Black beans, chickpeas, or kidney beans - exceptional sources of protein and fiber.

2. Healthy Fats and Oils

> **Extra Virgin Olive Oil:** Heart-friendly monounsaturated fats for cooking.
> **Avocado Oil:** High smoke point, suitable for high-temperature cooking.
> **Nuts and Seeds:** Almonds, walnuts, chia seeds, flaxseeds - abundant in omega-3 fatty acids.

3. Flavor Amplifiers

- ➢ **Herbs and Spices:** Cumin, turmeric, paprika, cinnamon - adding depth without added calories.
- ➢ **Low-Sodium Vegetable Broth:** Adaptable for soups, stews, and sauces.
- ➢ **Vinegars:** Balsamic, apple cider, or red wine vinegar - fantastic for dressings and marinades.

4. Canned and Jarred Essentials

- ➢ **Canned Tomatoes:** Enhances sauces and stews.
- ➢ **Tuna or Salmon:** Omega-3 rich, convenient protein sources.
- ➢ **Natural Nut Butters:** Peanut or almond butter - rich in protein and healthy fats.

5. Miscellaneous Pantry Staples

- ➢ **Whole Wheat Pasta or Substitutes:** Providing diversity in meal options.
- ➢ **Dark Chocolate:** An occasional treat - high cocoa content, lower sugar.
- ➢ **Honey or Maple Syrup:** Natural sweeteners to limit refined sugars.

5:2. ORGANIZATIONAL TIPS FOR KEEPING THE PANTRY WELL-STOCKED AND EFFICIENT.

Maintaining a well-ordered pantry streamlines cooking and ensures ingredient accessibility.
Here are some tips to keep your pantry well-organized and efficiently stocked:

1. **Group Similar Items:**
   Organize items by category to establish a structured arrangement. Sort grains, oils, canned goods, spices, and other ingredients into specific sections. This systematic approach simplifies access and enhances convenience during meal preparation.

2. **Optimize Shelf Usage:**
   Strategically position frequently used items within easy reach. Arrange essentials at eye level to avoid overcrowding and facilitate hassle-free cooking. Utilize vertical space for smaller items or spices to maximize storage efficiency.

3. **Label and Date Items:**
Clearly label containers, jars, or bins for quick identification of contents. Add purchase or expiry dates to ensure freshness. This labeling practice aids in utilizing items before they expire, preventing unnecessary waste.

4. **Conduct Regular Inventory Checks:**
Periodically assess your pantry supplies. Maintain a checklist to monitor items that require restocking. This routine review helps uphold a consistent inventory of essential ingredients, preventing shortages.

5. **Transparent Storage:**
Store commonly used items like grains, lentils, or nuts in transparent containers. Transparent jars or bins enable easy visibility, allowing you to gauge quantities and promptly replenish supplies when needed.

6. **Ensure Proper Storage:**
   Seal bags or containers effectively to preserve ingredient freshness. Store items in a cool, dry environment to maintain their quality. Consider airtight containers for ingredients susceptible to spoilage, such as flour, nuts, or seeds.

7. **Personalize Organization:**
   Customize your pantry layout based on your cooking routines. Arrange items according to meal preparations or cooking styles. For instance, group ingredients by cuisine or meal categories to streamline accessibility.

8. **Categorization of Supplies:**
   Group items by category (grains, oils, canned goods) for easy access.

9. **Optimal Shelf Placement:**
   Keep frequently used items at eye level for convenience.

Implementing these organization methods helps sustain a well-arranged and fully stocked pantry. It streamlines meal preparation, reduces clutter, and ensures ingredients are readily available, ultimately enhancing efficiency in the kitchen.

CHAPTER SIX

A 60-DAY MEAL PLAN

6:0. 60-DAY MEAL PLAN WITH DIVERSE, FLAVORFUL AND EASY-TO-FOLLOW RECIPES

Creating a 60-Day Meal plan with a variety of flavorful and straightforward recipes is an excellent way to embrace a heart-healthy lifestyle. This meal plan will offer diversity, ensuring that each day's meals are not only nutritious but also enjoyable to prepare and consume.

6:1. BALANCED BREAKFAST IDEAS

Breakfast is more than just the start of your day; it's the catalyst for your energy and vitality. Explore a range of balanced breakfast options that not only promise delectable flavors but also infuse your day with essential nourishment.

1. Hearty Oatmeal Bowls:

Delight in the comfort of hearty oatmeal bowls, uniting the wholesomeness of oats with an explosion of delectable toppings. Customize your oats with a medley of fruits like succulent strawberries, creamy bananas, or juicy blueberries. Sprinkle on crunchy almonds or walnuts for texture, and add a drizzle of honey or a dollop of yogurt for a touch of sweetness.

2. Yogurt Parfaits:

Indulge in luscious yogurt parfaits harmonizing the tang of yogurt with the sweetness of fruits and the crunch of granola. Layer your favorite yogurt with an array of fresh fruits like vibrant berries, sliced kiwi, or cubes of ripe mango. Top it off with a generous sprinkle of granola for an enticing blend of textures and flavors.

3. Nut Butter Toasts:

Elevate your morning toast by spreading sumptuous nut butter on whole-grain bread. Select from an array of almond, peanut, or cashew butter, and adorn it with sliced bananas, a drizzle of honey, or a dusting of cinnamon for a fulfilling and invigorating breakfast delight.

4. Veggie-Packed Egg Scrambles:

Relish the goodness of scrambled eggs packed with an array of vibrant vegetables. Create a colorful fusion of bell peppers, spinach, tomatoes, and mushrooms, fold them into beaten eggs, and cook until fluffy. Serve it alongside whole-grain toast or wrapped in a tortilla for a satisfying and nutritious breakfast.

5. Smoothie Bowls:

Plunge into refreshing smoothie bowls brimming with nutrients and bursting with flavors. Blend an assortment of fruits like zesty pineapple, succulent mango, and assorted berries with Greek yogurt or almond milk. Pour the smoothie into a bowl and top it with granola, shredded coconut, or nuts for added texture and zest.

6. Whole-Grain Pancakes or Waffles:

Indulge guilt-free in whole-grain pancakes or waffles crafted from whole-grain flour, complemented by mashed bananas or unsweetened applesauce for natural sweetness. Crown them with fresh fruit, a dollop of yogurt, or a drizzle of pure maple syrup for a delightful breakfast indulgence.

These diverse breakfast ideas promise a fusion of flavors, textures, and crucial nutrients, setting the stage for a dynamic and invigorating day. Revitalize your mornings with these delightful and nourishing breakfast selections.

6:2. NUTRIENT-PACKED LUNCHES

Lunchtime calls for fueling your energy levels. This meal plan presents a spectrum of fulfilling and nutrient-packed lunch options. Explore vibrant salads crowned with protein-rich toppings, wholesome whole-grain wraps crammed with veggies and lean proteins, or hearty grain bowls tantalizing your taste buds with an array of flavors and textures.

1. Vibrant Quinoa Salad Bowls:

Savor the abundance of a vibrant quinoa salad bowl brimming with nutrients and lively flavors. Combine cooked quinoa with an array of freshly diced vegetables like vibrant bell peppers, juicy cherry tomatoes, crisp cucumber slices, and vibrant leafy greens such as spinach or kale. Drizzle a zesty vinaigrette or a refreshing citrus dressing for a revitalizing lunch experience.

2. Protein-Loaded Veggie Wraps:

Bundle up a protein-rich meal by layering a whole-grain tortilla with a spread of hummus or Greek yogurt and an assortment of raw veggies—crisp shredded carrots, sliced bell peppers, cucumbers, and leafy greens. Amp up the protein with grilled tofu, chicken, or turkey and roll it into a satisfying, nutrient-packed wrap.

3. Wholesome Grain Harvest Bowls:

Craft nourishing grain bowls by blending whole grains, lean proteins, and an array of vibrant veggies. Mix brown rice or barley with roasted or sautéed vegetables like broccoli, cauliflower, carrots, and incorporate grilled salmon, boiled eggs, or chickpeas. Sprinkle seeds or nuts generously for an added texture and nutritional boost.

4. Flavorful Veggie Stir-Fry Feasts:

Create a symphony of colors and flavors with a delightful vegetable stir-fry featuring an assortment of bell peppers, crunchy snow peas, tender broccoli florets, and earthy mushrooms. Stir-fry these vegetables with aromatic ginger, garlic, and a light, flavorful sauce served alongside brown rice or whole-grain noodles.

5. Hearty Lentil Soups:

Relish in a comforting bowl of hearty lentil soup packed with proteins and fibers. Simmer lentils with fragrant herbs, onions, carrots, and celery for a rich and nutrient-dense soup. Elevate it further with the addition of spinach or kale, indulging in each spoonful paired with a slice of wholesome, whole-grain bread.

6. Abundant Buddha Bowls:

Craft an abundant Buddha bowl, featuring a base of quinoa or brown rice, adorned with a medley of roasted or raw vegetables, slices of creamy avocado, and a protein source like grilled tofu or shredded chicken. Crown it with a luscious drizzle of creamy tahini or avocado dressing for a deeply satisfying meal.

These nutrient-enriched lunch ideas are a symphony of flavors and nutrients, promising a vibrant midday meal that not only satisfies taste buds but also fuels your body with essential nourishment to seize the day.

6:3. WHOLESOME DINNER DELIGHTS

As the day winds down, indulge in fulfilling and wholesome dinners. Unearth flavorsome recipes like oven-baked fish complemented by roasted veggies, comforting soups bustling with an assortment of vegetables and legumes, or mouthwatering stir-fries bursting with colorful veggies and lean proteins, wrapping up your day on a satisfying note.

1. Flavorful Herb-Rubbed Baked Fish with Seasonal Roasted Vegetables:

Experience the delight of succulent baked fish adorned with a harmonious blend of herbs and spices. Select your preferred fish, season it generously, and bake it to perfection. Pair this exquisite dish with a symphony of roasted seasonal vegetables like caramelized carrots, grilled zucchini, and vibrant bell peppers, adding depth and wholesomeness to your dinner table.

2. Vibrant Vegetable Stir-Fries:

Embark on a flavorful journey with vegetable stir-fries boasting an eclectic mix of crunchy and colorful vegetables. Sauté an ensemble of vegetables—crisp bell peppers, broccoli florets, snap peas, earthy mushrooms—enhanced with aromatic garlic, ginger, and a touch of low-sodium soy sauce or teriyaki essence. Serve this aromatic medley with nutty brown rice or nutty quinoa for a gratifying meal.

3. Protein-Packed Salads with Grilled Chicken or Tofu:

Craft nourishing salads that offer a medley of textures and flavors by combining leafy greens with grilled chicken or tofu, an assortment of vibrant vegetables, and a sprinkle of wholesome seeds or nuts. Drizzle with a tangy vinaigrette or a velvety yogurt-based dressing for a lusciously wholesome and satiating dinner ensemble.

4. Hearty Nutrient-Infused Veggie Soups:

Cozy up with a heartwarming bowl of vegetable soup teeming with an assortment of nutritious veggies like sweet carrots, fragrant celery, verdant spinach, and robust legumes. Season it with a delightful medley of herbs and spices for a richly flavored and nourishing dinner experience that provides both comfort and healthfulness.

5. Wholesome Whole-Grain Pasta Varieties with Garden-Fresh Additions:

Delight in the wholesomeness of whole-grain pasta intertwined with a spectrum of nutritious enhancements. Toss whole-grain pasta in a homemade tomato sauce generously filled with an array of vegetables like earthy mushrooms, succulent bell peppers, and vibrant spinach. Finish with a sprinkle of grated cheese or a bouquet of fresh herbs for a flavorsome and nutrition-packed dinner treat.

6. Savory Bean-Centric Creations:

Indulge in the inviting flavors of bean-based culinary creations such as robust chili, aromatic bean stew, or tantalizing bean-based curries. Merge an assortment of beans—luscious black beans, creamy kidney beans, or versatile chickpeas—with fragrant spices, garden-fresh vegetables, and aromatic herbs for a hearty, protein-rich dinner that embodies both wholesomeness and gustatory pleasure.

These thoughtfully curated dinner ideas combine flavors and nutrients, ensuring that your evenings culminate in not just delectable but also nutritionally fulfilling experiences, culminating your day with wholesome and delightful culinary delights.

6:4. SMART AND HEALTHY SNACK CHOICES

Between meals, relish nutritious yet delectable snacks to keep those hunger pangs at bay. Tantalize your taste buds with homemade energy bars, crisp vegetable sticks dipped in luscious hummus, or revitalizing fruit salads - perfect guilt-free indulgences for those midday cravings.

1. Crispy Veggie Sticks with Homemade Dips:

Dive into a world of nutrient-packed goodness with a variety of fresh, crunchy vegetable sticks paired with vibrant homemade dips. Embrace the snap of carrot batons, bell pepper strips, cucumber spears, and celery sticks served alongside homemade hummus or a zesty Greek yogurt dip. These vitamin-rich delights offer a refreshing and healthy snack option.

2. Wholesome Homemade Energy Boosts:

Elevate your snack game with homemade energy bars that fuse together a medley of nutritious ingredients. Combine hearty oats, an assortment of nuts, nutrient-rich seeds, and dried fruits held together by natural sweeteners like honey or dates. These bars not only pack a punch of energy-boosting nutrients but also provide a delightful snack for your active days.

3. Vibrant Fresh Fruit Medley or Mixed Fruit Salad:

Treat your taste buds to a kaleidoscope of flavors with a vibrant medley of fresh fruits or a mosaic-like fruit salad. Enjoy a fusion of seasonal fruits such as succulent berries, juicy melons, zesty citrus fruits, and exotic tropical delights, abundant in vitamins, antioxidants, and natural sweetness—a refreshing and hydrating snack brimming with healthful advantages.

4. Nutrient-Packed Nut Butter Pairings:

Satisfy your snack cravings with the delicious pairing of creamy nut butter on whole-grain crackers or apple wedges. Select from a variety of nut butters—almond, peanut, or cashew—spread generously on whole-grain crackers or paired with apple slices. This union offers a satiating blend of protein, healthy fats, and fiber, ensuring a fulfilling and nutritious snack.

5. Indulgent Greek Yogurt Parfaits:

Delight in luxurious Greek yogurt parfaits layered with a riot of antioxidant-rich berries and crispy granola. Revel in the creamy texture of Greek yogurt infused with the natural sweetness of fresh berries and the gratifying crunch of granola. These protein-packed parfaits make for a nutrient-dense snack, perfect for satisfying your midday cravings.

6. Savory Oven-Roasted Seasoned Chickpeas:

Embark on a flavorful journey with savory oven-roasted chickpeas seasoned with a delightful blend of spices like paprika, cumin, or garlic powder. Roasted to a satisfying crunch, these seasoned chickpeas offer a deliciously savory and protein-rich snack option—a wholesome treat that's both satisfying and nutritious.

By opting for these intelligent and nutritious snack options, you'll satisfy those cravings while ensuring your body receives a plethora of essential nutrients, fostering a balanced and healthful approach to snacking.

6:5. DAILY GUIDANCE AND TIMELY SCHEDULES

Detailed daily schedules accompany the meal plan, guiding newcomers through this heart-healthy journey. These schedules meticulously outline each day's meals, providing straightforward instructions, enabling beginners to navigate their way through this nutritious culinary experience seamlessly.

1. Morning Rituals: Power Up Your Day

Begin your mornings with purposeful rituals that fuel your energy and set the pace for the day. Embrace activities like mindfulness exercises, gentle stretches, or an energizing yoga routine to awaken your mind and body. Enjoy a balanced and nutritious breakfast to kickstart your day with vitality and focus.

2. Meal Planning and Culinary Prep: Organize Your Dietary Journey

Allocate time for planning and preparing meals to ensure a wholesome and diverse diet. Designate a specific day for crafting a weekly meal plan with an array of heart-healthy options. Dedicate moments for grocery shopping, ingredient prepping, and perhaps even batch cooking for added convenience during busy stretches.

3. Hydration and Active Revival: Recharge Throughout the Day

Maintain hydration by drinking water regularly to keep your body refreshed. Embed active breaks into your daily schedule—take brief walks, practice desk exercises, or stretch to rejuvenate both your mind and body, especially during extended periods of desk-bound work or inactivity.

4. Mindful Eating: Relish Each Nourishing Bite

Cultivate mindfulness while consuming your meals by immersing yourself in the textures, tastes, and satisfaction derived from each bite. Eliminate distractions during meals, chew slowly, and relish every morsel. Tune into your body's hunger and fullness cues, fostering a harmonious relationship with food.

5. Evening Relaxation: Unwind and Ease into Nighttime

Design an evening routine that facilitates relaxation and prepares you for a restful night's sleep. Engage in calming activities such as unwinding with a book, practicing gentle yoga, or indulging in moments of meditation to alleviate stress. Reduce screen exposure before bedtime to enhance sleep quality and overall well-being.

6. Consistent Self-Check: Track Progress and Adapt

Incorporate regular check-ins to monitor your progress and fine-tune your routines. Reflect on your habits, identify obstacles faced, acknowledge achievements, and tweak your strategies to realign with your heart-healthy objectives.

A meticulously structured daily routine, infused with timely practices, lays the groundwork for maintaining consistency and navigating the path towards enhanced heart health. Embrace these practices to establish a harmonious, purposeful routine that nurtures your holistic well-being.

6:6. DETAILED DAILY SCHEDULES TO GUIDE BEGINNERS THROUGH THE MEAL PLAN

The cornerstone of successful meal planning, particularly for Beginners starting a heart-healthy journey, hinges on crafting intricate daily schedules. These schedules function as a well-organized blueprint, dissecting a comprehensive two-month meal plan into an assortment of varied, delectable recipes.

Their purpose is to keep newcomers aligned by furnishing detailed, sequential directives for each day's meals, focusing on nutritional equilibrium, diverse ingredients, and uncomplicated cooking techniques.

From invigorating breakfasts to fulfilling dinners and strategic snack selections, these schedules present an array of enticing choices.

They are meticulously structured, unambiguous, and supplemented with itemized shopping lists, instilling newcomers with the confidence to embrace and perpetuate a wholesome lifestyle.

Embark on this 60-day meal plan and immerse yourself in an enriching and flavorsome culinary voyage while nurturing your heart health.

Each day's meals are carefully crafted, promising a wide array of flavorful, diverse, and effortlessly prepared recipes, ensuring a satisfying and wholesome dietary adventure.

CHAPTER SEVEN

FAQ HIGHLIGHTS

7:1. ADDRESSING COMMON QUESTIONS ABOUT HEART-HEALTHY COOKING

1. What constitutes a diet that is heart-healthy?

Eating nutrient-dense meals including fruits, vegetables, whole grains, lean meats, and healthy fats is usually part of a heart-healthy diet. Limiting processed meals, saturated fats, salt, and added sugars is another aspect of it.

2. Are all fats detrimental to heart health?

Not every fat is bad for you. When ingested in moderation, healthy fats—such as those in nuts, seeds, avocados, and fatty fish—can promote heart health.

3. How much salt is appropriate for a diet that promotes heart health?

For most individuals, a daily salt consumption of no more than 2,300 mg is advised. Some medical disorders, however, can require even lower consumption.

4. How can physical activity affect heart health?

Exercise on a regular basis is essential for heart health. Spending at least 150 minutes a week exercising, such as brisk walking, swimming, or cycling, can have a major positive impact on heart health.

5. Can a diet that promotes heart health be pleasant and enjoyable?

A tasty, varied diet may be heart-healthy. Meals may be flavored and healthful by experimenting with different recipes, adding vibrant foods, and utilizing herbs and spices.

6. What are some ways to include more fruits and veggies in my meals?

Make an effort to include fruits in your morning meals, eat salads or soups made mostly of vegetables at lunch, and make sure that veggies are a big part of your dinner plate. A great method to enhance consumption is to have fruit and vegetable snacks.

7. Are there any particular foods that are better for heart health to avoid?

In general, it is advisable to restrict or avoid foods high in trans fats, processed sweets, and excessive salt when following a heart-healthy diet. Reducing the amount of processed and fried meals consumed is also advantageous.

7:2. TROUBLESHOOTING GUIDE FOR BEGINNER COOKS FACING CHALLENGES IN THE KITCHEN

1. Recipes Yielding Unexpected Results

Solution: Ensure precise measurements and adherence to recipes. Start with straightforward recipes before advancing to more complex ones. Refer to trustworthy sources for recipes.

2. Time Management Hiccups

Solution: Plan meals in advance, prep ingredients early, and prioritize tasks. Employ timers or user-friendly cooking apps for efficient time management.

3. Overcooking or Undercooking Dishes

Solution: Invest in a reliable kitchen thermometer. Follow recommended cooking durations, relying on visual and textural cues for dish readiness. Practice enhances judgment.

4. Lack of Flavor in Dishes

Solution: Experiment with diverse herbs, spices, and seasonings. Taste food while cooking and make adjustments as needed. Understand how various spices complement different dishes.

5. Difficulty in Juggling Multiple Tasks

Solution: Commence with simpler recipes having fewer components. Organize tasks, prep ingredients beforehand, and concentrate on one task at a time. Confidence in multitasking develops gradually.

6. Unorganized Kitchen Setup

Solution: Maintain a tidy workspace by cleaning as you progress. Arrange utensils and ingredients beforehand. Wash dishes simultaneously while cooking.

7. Feeling Overwhelmed by Complex Recipes or Techniques

Solution: Initiate cooking with basic recipes and methods. Watch tutorials, peruse beginner-friendly cookbooks, or enroll in online classes to ease into complex techniques gradually.

8. Difficulty Adapting Recipes for Dietary Preferences or Restrictions

Solution: Familiarize yourself with ingredient substitutes and modifications. Explore specialized cookbooks or websites catering to specific dietary needs. Experiment with alternative ingredients.

9. Handling Kitchen Accidents or Errors

Solution: Stay composed and learn from mistakes. Keep essential first aid supplies easily accessible. Be informed about emergency protocols in case of unforeseen accidents.

10. Burnt or Food Sticking to Pans

> **Solution:** Manage heat levels effectively, opt for non-stick cookware, and use oil/butter as required. Use appropriate utensils for stirring or flipping to prevent food from adhering.

Remember, everyone encounters kitchen challenges, particularly when starting out.

Patience, practice, and an eagerness to learn from errors are essential for enhancing culinary prowess!

CHAPTER EIGHT

2000+ DAYS OF DIVERSE RECIPES

8:1. A VAST SELECTION OF OVER 2000 RECIPES SPANNING VARIOUS CUISINES AND FLAVORS

Developing an extensive library housing more than 2000 recipes is akin to embarking on a global culinary expedition. This gastronomic anthology traverses an array of culinary traditions and tastes, presenting a treasury of epicurean adventures.

This extensive compendium delves into a myriad of culinary cultures, capturing flavors from around the globe.

From the aromatic spice blends of Indian gastronomy to the indulgent depths of Italian pasta concoctions, the meticulous artistry behind Japanese sushi, the vibrant zest of Mexican taco assemblies, and the hearty goodness found in Middle Eastern stews, this mosaic of recipes embarks on a culinary voyage spanning continents.

Within this compendium of 2000+ recipes, one can indulge in a kaleidoscope of tastes and cooking techniques, catering to an array of palates and dietary requirements. Embracing options from vegetarian or vegan dishes to protein-rich concoctions, gluten-free or dairy-free delicacies, and sumptuous dessert creations, this diverse compendium caters to every culinary inclination and nutritional necessity.

Each recipe is a tale woven from a unique tapestry of ingredients, methods, and cultural influences, presenting an opportunity to dive into the world of culinary arts. It's an expedition for learning, experimentation, and the crafting of meals that tantalize the senses while narrating tales of cultural heritage through gastronomy.

Moreover, this extensive compilation serves as an invaluable guide for novices and expert chefs alike, presenting an extensive array of choices to explore and hone culinary expertise. It embodies the infinite potential of culinary artistry, unveiling the limitless prospects and innovation that can be expressed through food.

Ultimately, assembling over 2000 recipes from diverse cuisines and flavor palettes transcends mere quantity; it's an ode to the rich tapestry of diversity, the thrill of culinary exploration, and the ability to invite the world's culinary heritage into one's kitchen for an experience meant to be relished and shared.

8:2. CATEGORIZATION BASED ON MEAL TYPES, INGREDIENTS, AND COOKING DIFFICULTY LEVELS

1. MEAL TYPES:

Breakfast:

Presenting a wide array of revitalizing and nourishing recipes, such as oatmeal variations, smoothie bowls bursting with fresh fruits, and savory breakfast wraps filled with wholesome ingredients. This category also encompasses an assortment of invigorating morning beverages, including energizing smoothies, rejuvenating teas, or aromatic coffees.

Lunch:

Curating an extensive selection of diverse midday meal options, from vibrant and hearty salads packed with nutritious greens to soul-soothing soups, sandwiches filled with delectable ingredients, and grain bowls brimming with satisfying flavors. Lunch recipes are carefully crafted for quick preparation without compromising on taste and balance.

Dinner:

Offering a diverse culinary landscape with an array of comforting and flavorful dinner choices, including comforting stews, sumptuous pasta dishes, nourishing casseroles, perfectly grilled meats, seafood extravaganzas, and innovative vegetable-centric mains. These recipes cater to varied palates and preferences, ensuring a delightful dinner experience.

Snacks:

Providing an assortment of tantalizing quick bites or light nibbles, such as energy-boosting bars, delightful dips, finger-licking finger foods, or small bites perfect for satiating between-meal cravings without compromising on healthiness.

Desserts:

Featuring a tempting collection of sweet indulgences, ranging from decadent cakes, irresistible cookies, and flaky pies to healthier dessert alternatives like fruit-based creations, luscious puddings, or tantalizing frozen delights. These recipes satisfy the sweet tooth while offering various health-conscious options.

2. INGREDIENTS:

Vegetarian:

Showcasing an array of vibrant and flavorful recipes crafted without meat or fish, emphasizing the goodness of plant-based dishes loaded with an assortment of vibrant vegetables, legumes, grains, and an abundance of seasonal fruits.

Vegan:

Curating a diverse set of recipes entirely excluding animal products, showcasing ingenious plant-based alternatives and inventive adaptations of traditional dishes, ranging from hearty mains to tantalizing desserts, ensuring a delightful exploration of cruelty-free culinary experiences.

Gluten-Free:

Providing an extensive array of recipes eliminating gluten-containing grains like wheat, barley, and rye, perfect for individuals with gluten sensitivities or celiac disease, offering delicious alternatives without compromising on taste or quality.

Dairy-Free:

Presenting a variety of delectable recipes free from dairy products, suitable for those with lactose intolerance or dietary preferences steering clear of dairy, offering flavorful and wholesome alternatives for cooking and baking.

Low-Carb:

Featuring a curated selection of recipes focused on reducing carbohydrate intake while incorporating higher protein and healthy fats, ideal for individuals following low-carb diets, ensuring satisfying and nutritious meals without sacrificing taste or variety.

3. COOKING DIFFICULTY LEVELS:

- **Beginner:**
Offering a diverse range of straightforward and uncomplicated recipes tailored for novice cooks or those seeking easy-to-follow dishes to develop culinary skills and gain confidence in the kitchen.

- **Intermediate:**
Providing recipes with moderate complexity, presenting an opportunity for enhancing cooking skills and techniques, suitable for individuals with some culinary experience seeking new challenges.

- **Advanced:** Showcasing intricate and sophisticated recipes that demand expert culinary techniques, perfect for seasoned cooks eager to embark on gastronomic adventures and master challenging culinary endeavors.

These extensive categories serve as a comprehensive guide, facilitating effortless navigation through an expansive repertoire of recipes.

Tailored to suit varying tastes, dietary preferences, and cooking expertise, this curated selection simplifies the culinary journey, ensuring a delightful exploration of diverse cuisines and flavors.

8:3. EMPHASIS ON VARIETY TO KEEP MEALS EXCITING AND ENJOYABLE

1. Culinary Global Voyage:
Explore a multitude of international cuisines, from Thai and Italian to Mexican and Indian. Each cuisine boasts distinct spices, herbs, and cooking methods, enriching meals with diversity and excitement.

2. Seasonal Gastronomic Journey:

Embrace seasonal produce, celebrating the unique flavors and textures offered throughout the year. Adapting recipes based on seasonal ingredients ensures freshness and introduces a fascinating culinary diversity.

3. Textural Symphony:

Infuse dishes with diverse textures—marry crispness with creaminess or add chewy or crunchy elements to softer dishes. This textural interplay elevates the dining experience with unexpected delights.

4. Artistic Plating:

Craft visually appealing dishes by integrating an array of colorful ingredients. Vibrant plates featuring a kaleidoscope of fruits and veggies offer not just visual allure but also a plethora of nutrients and tastes.

5. Innovative Culinary Techniques:

Experiment with various cooking methods like grilling, roasting, steaming, or braising. Each technique accentuates unique flavors and textures, bringing depth and intrigue to meals.

6. Fusion Fusion:

Combine elements from diverse culinary traditions to create fusion dishes. This imaginative blend infuses excitement by harmonizing the best of different cooking styles into one distinctive meal.

7. Thematic Dining:

Establish themed meal nights, such as Taco Tuesdays or Meatless Mondays. This introduces anticipation and culinary adventure, allowing for exploration and variety within a specific theme.

8. Exploration of Ingredients:

Regularly experiment with new and unconventional ingredients. From exotic fruits to unique spices, the introduction of novel ingredients adds freshness and excitement to cooking.

9. Heritage-Inspired Delights:

Incorporate traditional family recipes or dishes from cultural backgrounds. Sharing these recipes not only adds sentimental value but also injects meals with authenticity and diversity.

10. Dynamic Menu Rotation:

Keep menus lively by rotating dishes on a weekly or monthly basis. Blend new recipes with cherished classics to sustain variety and prevent meal monotony.

Through an emphasis on diverse ingredients, cooking techniques, and thoughtful meal planning, every dining occasion becomes an enjoyable exploration of culinary delight and cultural richness.

CHAPTER NINE

CONCLUSION

9:1. SUMMARIZING THE KEY TAKEAWAYS FROM THE COOKBOOK

A cookbook functions as an extensive manual, offering an array of valuable insights and practical wisdom for cooking enthusiasts.

Below is an elaborated overview highlighting the main takeaways:

1. Cooking Basics and Techniques:

Cookbooks serve as educational tools, imparting fundamental cooking skills like precise knife handling, temperature control, and safe food preparation. They introduce core techniques such as frying, baking, roasting, and stewing, laying a strong groundwork for newcomers while refining abilities for seasoned chefs.

2. Diverse Array of Recipes:

A cookbook houses a broad range of recipes spanning various cuisines, meal categories, and occasions. It boasts breakfast suggestions, appetizers, main courses, side dishes, desserts, and beverages, catering to a wide spectrum of tastes and inclinations.

3. Emphasis on Healthy Eating and Nutrition:

Many cookbooks prioritize health, advocating for well-balanced meals featuring whole grains, lean proteins, good fats, and an abundance of fruits and vegetables. They often spotlight the nutritional advantages of specific ingredients, guiding readers towards better dietary choices.

4. Innovative Cooking Techniques:

Certain cookbooks introduce inventive cooking methods, unique ingredient pairings, or alternative substitutes, encouraging culinary experimentation and imaginative approaches in the kitchen.

5. Meal Preparation Strategies:
Cookbooks offer insights into efficient meal planning, guidance on batch cooking, and tips for meal prepping, simplifying meal preparation, especially for those with hectic schedules.

6. Insights into Culture and Tradition:
Through recipes from diverse cultures, cookbooks provide insights into varied culinary traditions, the backstory of classic dishes, and how food acts as a cultural unifier across global communities.

7. Adaptability to Dietary Requirements:
Acknowledging varied dietary needs, many cookbooks feature recipes tailored to specific preferences or limitations, such as vegetarian, vegan, gluten-free, or low-carb diets, ensuring inclusivity and flexibility.

8. Advocacy for Holistic Wellness:

Beyond recipes, cookbooks promote overall well-being by advocating healthy lifestyle choices. They might include sections on physical fitness, stress management, or mindfulness, highlighting the significance of a well-rounded life.

9. Celebration of Culinary Experience:

Cookbooks celebrate the joy of cooking, prompting individuals to relish the cooking process, experiment with flavors, and create memorable meals to share with loved ones.

10. Continuous Learning and Inspiration:

Serving as an ever-present resource, cookbooks inspire ongoing learning, experimentation, and growth in the culinary world, nurturing a lifelong passion for cooking and exploration in the kitchen.

In essence, a cookbook is more than a mere compilation of recipes. It evolves into a companion, mentor, and a wellspring of inspiration, enriching the cooking journey and fostering a deeper appreciation for the art and delight of cooking.

9:2. ENCOURAGEMENT AND MOTIVATION TO CONTINUE THE JOURNEY TOWARD HEART-HEALTHY COOKING

1. Acknowledge Achievements:

Recognize even the smallest milestones. Encourage readers to applaud each step toward embracing a heart-healthy lifestyle, whether it's preparing a wholesome meal, experimenting with a fresh recipe, or altering dietary habits positively.

2. Community Involvement:

Stress the importance of building connections or finding support. Urge readers to engage with others on a similar path, exchange culinary experiences, share recipes, and provide mutual encouragement and motivation.

3. Practical Goal-Setting:

Help readers set practical objectives. Encourage them to define clear, attainable goals, such as integrating more vegetables into daily meals, lowering sodium intake, or committing to a specific number of heart-healthy dishes weekly.

4. Informative Insights:

Empower readers with knowledge. Offer informative content detailing the advantages of heart-healthy eating, the impact of diverse ingredients on cardiovascular health, and the science behind making nutritious dietary choices.

5. Diverse Culinary Exploration:

Foster culinary curiosity. Encourage readers to diversify their culinary endeavors by exploring new ingredients, cuisines, and cooking styles. Highlight the pleasure of discovering delectable yet heart-conscious recipes.

6. Incremental Progress:

Highlight the value of gradual change. Remind readers that small, consistent changes over time can lead to substantial improvements in health rather than striving for absolute perfection.

7. Mindful Eating Practices:

Advocate for mindful consumption. Encourage readers to relish each bite, consume meals slowly, and be mindful of hunger and satiety signals. Emphasize the satisfaction derived from mindful eating.

8. Adaptability and Openness:

Stress the importance of adaptability. Encourage readers to be open to adjusting recipes, incorporating substitutions, and accommodating personal preferences, understanding these are integral parts of the journey.

9. Self-Care and Equilibrium:

Advocate for holistic well-being. Emphasize the significance of balance in life, including ample rest, stress management, regular physical activity, and nurturing positive mental health alongside dietary changes.

10. Share Inspiring Narratives:

Present stories of success. Highlight real-life experiences of individuals who have embraced heart-healthy cooking, showcasing their positive well-being transformations. These narratives can serve as potent motivational tools for readers.

9:3. CLOSING REMARKS AND BEST WISHES FOR A HEALTHIER LIFESTYLE

This journey is about much more than the food on your table; it's a vibrant celebration of life, deliberate choice, and the unadulterated thrill of tasting every distinct and mouth watering flavor life has to offer.

May you find great satisfaction in your quest for a healthier living with every step you take down this path. Savor every second you spend in the kitchen, whether it's investigating unknown and new ingredients with curiosity, experimenting with recipes without fear, or just enjoying the pure joy of creating culinary marvels.

I hope that your path to become an expert in heart-healthy cuisine will be an inspiration to you and everyone around you, both personally and professionally. Let what you learn inspire others to embrace the nutritious nature of whole foods and build a supportive community that is rooted in wellness and hope.

Celebrate all of your accomplishments, no matter how minor, enjoy the rainbow of tastes dancing on your palate, and cherish every delicious mouthful that demonstrates your commitment to become a better version of yourself.

Cheers to your continued success and my sincere hopes for endless happiness, excellent health, and an abundance of times filled with sustenance and delicious culinary adventures in the future. I wish you a life full of heart-healthy, meaningful experiences and intriguing discoveries! May your path be loaded with blessings!

Warm compliments and sincere support on your continued path to become a more vibrant, healthy, and contented version of yourself.

APPENDIX

COMPLEMENT SECTIONS TO HEART HEALTHY COOKBOOK:

1. Nutrition Overview:

A comprehensive overview of nutritional information corresponding to each recipe, featuring details on calories, macronutrient composition, and essential vitamins and minerals. This segment aims to provide a clear insight into the nutritional value of every dish.

2. Enhancing Culinary Skills:

Supplementary guidance and advanced tips that complement the basic cooking techniques highlighted in the primary sections. This appendix section aims to offer deeper insights into refining cooking prowess.

3. Ingredient Compendium:

An exhaustive compendium outlining all ingredients featured in the cookbook, complete with descriptions, alternative options, and nutritional advantages. This guide assists in recognizing and comprehending the components used in the recipes.

4. Meal Planning Frameworks:

Customizable templates or frameworks designed to align with the cookbook's recipes, aiding readers in structuring weekly or monthly meal plans efficiently, fostering a heart-healthy culinary journey.

5. Conversion Tables:

Convenient tables featuring conversions for measurements (e.g., cups to grams), temperature adjustments, and other essential culinary conversions, facilitating seamless recipe execution.

6. Recommended Culinary Tools:

Recommendations and insights into essential kitchen tools and equipment that can elevate the cooking experience and streamline the preparation of heart-healthy meals.

7. Ingredient Swapping Handbook:

Information on alternative ingredients and substitutions suited for specific dietary preferences or limitations, offering adaptability in recipe modification while upholding the focus on heart-healthy choices.

8. Exploring Advanced Techniques:

An advanced section showcasing complex cooking methods, intricate recipes, and culinary approaches for individuals seeking to advance their skills beyond beginner levels.

9. Efficient Meal Prep Strategies:

Detailed strategies and guides for effective meal preparation, including tips on bulk cooking, ingredient storage, and prepping elements in advance for heart-healthy meal preparation.

10. Community Connection Resources:
Insights into online forums, social media groups, or local cooking communities where readers can engage, exchange experiences, and seek further guidance or inspiration related to heart-healthy cooking.

THE END